# Reverse Diabetes

### 30 Best Superfoods to Prevent and Reverse Diabetes and 30 Worst Foods to Avoid

**INCLUDES OVER 30 SUPERFOOD DIABETES FRIENDLY RECIPES TO REGULATE INSULIN, CONTROL BLOOD SUGAR AND LOWER BLOOD PRESSURE**

Copyright © 2017 Kasia Roberts, RN

All Right Reserved.

# Disclaimer

The information in this book is not to be used as medical advice. The recipes should be used in combination with guidance from your physician. Please consult your physician before beginning any diet. It is especially important for those with diabetes, and those on medications to consult with their physician before making changes to their diet.

All rights reserved. No part of this publication or the information in it may be quoted from or reproduced in any form by means such as printing, scanning, photocopying or otherwise without prior written permission of the copyright holder.

Disclaimer and Terms of Use: Effort has been made to ensure that the information in this book is accurate and complete, however, the author and the publisher do not warrant the accuracy of the information, text and graphics contained within the book due to the rapidly changing nature of science, research, known and unknown facts and internet. The Author and the publisher do not hold any responsibility for errors, omissions or contrary interpretation of the subject matter herein. This book is presented solely for motivational and informational purposes only.

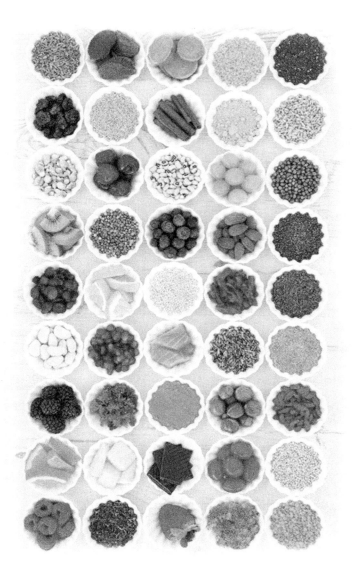

# Introduction

Receiving the type 2 diabetes diagnosis can feel like a death sentence—or, at least, an assurance that your entire life is about to change. But now that you know, once and for all, that your body doesn't make insulin well and thus cannot use glucose readily for fuel, you can begin to take action, every single day, to care for yourself, boost your longevity, promote stable blood sugar levels, and gravitate away from terrible diabetes symptoms. If you plan correctly, you can even lose weight and look your best, despite having this diagnosis. When you regularly include in your diet amazing foods that heal – food can be a powerful medicine.

This book enables you to take type 2 diabetes seriously. If you don't take action, by incorporating more superfoods into your diet—and eliminating those "other" foods that are making you sicker—you can ultimately have a heart attack or stroke, have eye problems, such as blindness, lose feeling in your feet, have gum and teeth problems, or even lose control of your kidneys.

Superfoods are foods found in nature that are incredibly healthy, containing antioxidants, vitamins, and minerals. These foods often decrease your risk of cancers, cardiovascular diseases, obesity, and countless other ailments. However, they're also essential for blood sugar stability, one thing that can lead to a better, simpler diabetic lifestyle.

Armed with 30 superfoods, including strawberries, broccoli, kale, salmon, and many others, you can begin to understand how these foods will alter your body on a cellular level and help you regulate your type 2 diabetes. The recipes, included in breakfast, lunch, and dinner chapters, are pulsing with vibrant superfoods, and also include nutritional information to help you keep on track, including carbohydrate count, fat count, and protein count. Best of all: each recipe contains only 15 grams of net carbohydrates per serving, meaning blood sugar spikes are a thing of the past.

An additional included chapter lists 30 foods, found so often in everyday life, that are exacerbating your type 2 diabetes symptoms, and are best avoided. Say goodbye to white bread, white pasta, and dreaded, sodium-rich fast food. They're destroying you, and literally cutting the length of your life.

Good luck on this journey. Find peace, improve your type 2 diabetes symptoms, and lose weight. Just because you've been diagnosed, doesn't mean your life is over.

# Table of Contents

**WHAT IS TYPE 2 DIABETES, AND WHO IS AT RISK?** ... 9

**DO I HAVE DIABETES? RECOGNIZING SIGNS AND SYMPTOMS** ... 19

**5 EASY STEPS TO REVERSE DIABETES SYMPTOMS** ... 28

**DIABETIC LIVING IN THE KITCHEN: SHOPPING LIST** ... 39

**TOP NATURAL REMEDIES, HERBS, AND VITAMINS** ... 50

**30 BEST SUPERFOODS TO COMBAT TYPE 2 DIABETES** ... 57

**30 WORST FOODS, BEST AVOIDED IF YOU HAVE DIABETES** ... 73

**LOW CARB SUPERFOOD BREAKFAST RECIPES** ... 93
   GREEN PERFECTION MATCHA BOWL ... 94
   CINNAMON APPLE FLAXSEED WAFFLES ... 96
   LOW CARB EGG WHITE OMELET ... 98
   LOW CARB CINNAMON "OATMEAL" ... 100
   HEALTHY MORNING MUFFINS ... 103
   BRITISH BLUEBERRY POPOVERS WITH FRUIT SALAD TOPPING ... 105
   LOW CARB COCONUT FLOUR GARLIC BAGELS ... 108
   KALE AND SWEET POTATO HASH ... 110
   QUINOA AND POMEGRANATE MORNING PORRIDGE ... 112
   SPINACH EGG WHITE QUICHE ... 114
   BREAKFAST SMOOTHIE - ALMOND MILK AND FLAX SEED SMOOTHIE ... 116
   BREAKFAST SMOOTHIE - SATISFYING RICE-BASED PROTEIN SHAKE ... 117

## LOW CARB SUPERFOOD LUNCH RECIPES ............ 119
FLAXSEED BREAD FOR HEALTHY, SUPERFOOD
SANDWICHES ............................................................. 120
AVOCADO AND CAPRESE SALAD ............................. 123
TUNA AND AVOCADO SALAD .................................. 125
VEGGIE SPAGHETTI SQUASH ................................... 127
CHICKPEA AND SALMON SALAD ............................. 130
LOW CARB MEXICAN SOUP IN THE SLOW COOKER ......... 132
TURKEY BACON BROCCOLI SALAD .......................... 134
BLACK BEAN AND CHICKEN SOUP ........................... 136
FLAXSEED TORTILLA TACOS ................................... 138
SUPERFOOD PUMPKIN SOUP .................................. 141

## LOW CARB SUPERFOOD DINNER RECIPES ........... 145
CURRIED CHICKEN AND VEGETABLES ..................... 146
PESKY PESTO CHICKEN WITH WALNUTS ................. 148
CHICKEN SHAWARMA WITH A LEMON AND BASIL GLAZE
............................................................................... 150
GARLIC SALMON WITH TOMATOES ........................ 153
ASIAN SALMON COATED WITH BLACK BEAN SAUCE ....... 155
LOW CARB, EASY SCALLOPS WITH VEGETABLE STEW .... 158
CAULIFLOWER PIZZA CRUST WITH VEGAN TOPPINGS .... 160
ASIAN ASPARAGUS AND TURKEY ............................ 163
WALNUT DINNER SALAD WITH FETA AND CRANBERRIES
............................................................................... 165
PISTACHIO AND KALE PESTO WITH HALIBUT .................. 167
EDAMAME VEGGIE BURGER ................................... 170
SKILLET WITH APPLES, CHICKEN, SWEET POTATOES, AND
BRUSSELS SPROUTS ................................................ 173
FRUIT CHUTNEY WITH SALMON CURRY ................. 175
TURKEY AND ESSENTIAL ROASTED ROOTS ............. 177

## CONCLUSION ............................................... 179

# What is Type 2 Diabetes, and Who is at Risk?

A diabetes epidemic is sweeping the world, forcing millions of individuals to look at the choices they make as the risk for chronic disease, stroke, heart attack, coma, and even death become increasingly higher. Diabetes is strongly correlated to the ways in which people in today's society live their lives and cannot be ignored any longer. We must deliberately choose a better way of life in order to be free of its symptoms and the required medication. We must seek a better course of action to create a more vibrant community that makes conscious lifestyle choices to regulate blood glucose levels and facilitate better physical and mental health.

At the core of diabetes lie your food choices. What you eat and how you eat it can dramatically define who you are on a cellular level. As your body metabolizes the food you ingest, it creates a steady stream of glucose that is meant to enter into your cells, fuel you with energy, and take you through the many adventures (or misadventures) of your life.

Unfortunately, what has been marketed so heartily throughout much of the western world—processed foods filled with junk additives, extra sugars, and mega bouts of sodium—is literally killing us. Note that diabetes is the seventh leading cause of death in the United States. We must retreat from these heavily marketed, shiny piles of fake food and fall back into our kitchens to create the vibrant, nutritive food our body so craves.

As we alter our lifestyle choices, cook healthy, nutritious meals, and become precise in the ways in which we live our lives, we can reverse diabetes symptoms. We can change the course of our lives. We can fuel ourselves with natural herbs, natural supplements, and essential superfoods to allow our bodies to do what they've been meaning to do all along: heal us, fuel us with good energy, and decrease the levels of inflammation currently demonizing our systems.

With this book in hand, you can change the course of your diabetic life. You can become free from your medication, from your fear of diabetes complications, and from your fear of high blood sugar spikes and decreases in the middle of the day. You can become a free-standing individual. Learn the secrets of reversing your diabetes, and anticipate a better, enriched future.

What if your body turned against you?

All your life, your body has been working to transfer the food you eat into energy, turning carbohydrates, fats, proteins, and other nutrients into fuel to keep you walking, talking, laughing, and feeling. Unfortunately, for millions of people around the world, their bodies don't continue this trajectory, due to many factors—many of them lifestyle-related. They become sick, remarkably so. And they must become extra diligent, with every morsel of food they put into their mouth, to ensure they don't die.

Yes: type 2 diabetes is a matter of life and death. But you can manage your type 2 diabetes by following a strict diet and focusing on superfoods, low carb diets, and other nutritional options.

## What Is Type 2 Diabetes?

Type 2 diabetes is a term that denotes the fact that your body doesn't use blood sugar, otherwise known as glucose, correctly anymore. Glucose is the energy your body stores in your muscle and tissue cells after you eat, and it's also the main source of energy for your brain.

When too much glucose builds up in your blood, your body grows increasingly insulin resistant. Your pancreas cannot create enough insulin to match the glucose in your bloodstream. As insulin is the hormone that forces your cells to accept glucose as fuel, your body grows increasingly "starved" of fuel.

As such, your body begins to breakdown, since your cells aren't receiving the energy they require. Often, people with diabetes lose a great deal of weight, just prior to their diagnosis. This is the body going into shock, the cells shrinking due to a loss of energy, and, despite the changing scale, shouldn't be seen as a good thing. Your body is simply unable to use the fuel you're feeding it.

As a result of this glucose buildup, your body becomes dehydrated. Your kidneys receive the brunt of all that glucose in your system, and it can't deal with it. The sugar within your urine ultimately draws water from your other cells as it passes through your bloodstream, causing you to urinate even more often. When a diabetic person becomes too dehydrated, they might develop a diabetic coma, otherwise known as hyperosmolar hyperglycemic non-ketotic syndrome. If this goes on too long, the high levels of glucose in your body can ultimately narrow your arteries, ultimately putting you at risk for stroke and heart attack.

Other symptoms of type 2 diabetes include the following: increased hunger, dry mouth, feeling increasingly tired, blurred vision, frequent infections, sudden and unexplainable weight loss or weight gain, sexual dysfunction, yeast infections, and many headaches.

## Who Is at Risk for Type 2 Diabetes?

Unfortunately, scientists don't have a full grasp of why some people develop diabetes, and others don't. In fact, you can develop type 2 diabetes at any age, even when you're younger. Generally speaking, however, type 2 diabetes strikes people who are middle-aged, do not consume a nutritious diet, and are overweight.

Look to the following factors, which often lead to diabetes:

You're overweight. If you have more fatty tissue on your body than you should, per your height and bone structure, your cells become more resistant to insulin, and thus won't allow glucose to be used as fuel.

You're not active. When you exercise, you're forcing your body to use up the glucose in your bloodstream, and also making your cells more sensitive to insulin. This means that your pancreas won't have to make as much insulin for your cells to react and take in glucose as fuel. This is good, since having too much insulin in your bloodstream can promote obesity and, naturally, diabetes.

Your family has a history of diabetes. If your parents, grandparents, or siblings have diabetes, then you have a higher chance of developing diabetes as well. Watch your food intake, and ensure that you exercise. You can outrun your genes.

You're Hispanic, Black, American Indian, or Asian-American. No one really knows the reason why, but these races are at a higher risk of developing diabetes, and of being overweight or obese. Again, you can outrun your genes.

You're getting up there in age. Of course, this could also be correlated with the fact that often, as you grow older, you don't exercise as much, you lose muscle, and you generally gravitate toward comfort foods. Make sure you pay attention to your food intake, even as you age, to rev your metabolism and fight against the onset of diabetes.

You have PCOS, or polycystic ovary syndrome. Some women who suffer from this disorder, which involves excessive hair growth, abnormal menstrual cycles, and obesity, are at a higher risk of developing diabetes.

You had or have gestational diabetes while you were pregnant. If you did, and you then gave birth to a baby that weighed more than nine pounds, you're at a higher risk of developing type 2 diabetes. Also, if you were overweight prior to the pregnancy, are over the age of 25, and have family members who suffered from gestational diabetes, you're at a greater risk.

Your cholesterol and triglyceride levels are off. According to scientists, we have two different kinds of cholesterol: high-density and low-density lipoproteins. In order to maintain your health, your high-density lipoproteins should be high. If they're low, then you're at a greater risk of developing type 2 diabetes. Furthermore, triglycerides, another fat in your bloodstream, should be low.

# The Future, If You Don't Make Changes

If you don't alter your lifestyle, post your diagnosis of your pre-diabetic or diabetic state, you're increasing your risk of cardiovascular disease, such as angina, heart attack, atherosclerosis, or the narrowing of the arteries, and stroke. With too much sugar in your bloodstream, you can burden the small blood vessels in your legs, ultimately causing numbness and nerve damage. Furthermore, diabetes can damage the blood vessels around your eyes, ultimately leading to blindness, glaucoma, or cataracts.

# Do I Have Diabetes? Recognizing Signs and Symptoms

So often, Type 2 diabetes is not diagnosed until the occurrence of health complications. The symptoms can be very gradual. Therefore, it's essential to know your body and listen for the following signs and symptoms. Remember that twenty-five percent of people with diabetes don't know they suffer from it.

Warning Signs and Symptoms

# 1. Frequent urination.

People with diabetes urinate often because glucose, or sugar, builds in the bloodstream as it cannot enter into the cells to be created into energy. As a result, the bloodstream's osmolality increases. Therefore, the bloodstream begins to yank fluid out of the bodily cells as it passes them on its way to the kidneys. This occurs because the bloodstream requires more water for balance between the "water" and the "glucose." The cells transmit this water. (Thus, diabetics become far thirstier.) As a result of this enhanced "water" blood, the kidney fills with extra fluid. The kidneys thus make more urine.

As a result, it's essential that people monitor their blood glucose levels to allow glucose to enter the cells and not dehydrate the body, pulling all the liquid out of the cells to be expelled through urination.

## 2. Incredible thirst.

As mentioned in the previous point, diabetics are much thirstier than normal because the blood glucose levels in the bloodstream force fluids from the cells. This increased load of liquid is sent to the kidneys and ultimately expelled. The cells require more hydration as a result, forcing diabetics to become thirstier.

## 3. Incredible hunger, despite eating.

The cells in the body cannot accept the glucose in the bloodstream because of the lack of insulin. As a result, the body cannot convert that glucose into energy, depleting the cells of their necessary boost. This formulates incredible hunger, even when eating and after eating.

Furthermore, many people with type 2 diabetes have a high level of insulin in the bloodstream—insulin that does not, of course, work properly. However, this increased level of insulin in the bloodstream tells the brain that the body is hungry.

## 4. Sudden and unforeseen weight loss.

People with type 2 diabetes cannot accept glucose into their cells. Therefore, the cells cannot store glucose as energy and must then look to stored fat for fuel. Furthermore, with the increased urination, the body begins to lose its calories quickly through the bloodstream and directly out through the kidneys.

5. Numb feet.

If diabetes goes unnoticed, it can ultimately damage some of the bodily nerves. The damage can either go completely unnoticed; alternately, it can bring pain or numbness to your feet and other extremities.

## 6. Greater risk of infection.

People with type 2 diabetes are at greater risk for infection. Most notably, women with type 2 diabetes have a greater risk of vaginal infections because their yeast and bacteria numbers multiply with the existence of greater blood sugar levels. Furthermore, many people suffer from feet infections because of damage to foot nerves, foot skin, and food blood vessels.

## 7. Inability to see well.

Occasionally, the lens of the eye—which is the membrane that alters the eye's focus, much like a mechanism on a camera—does not work properly in the first stages of type 2 diabetes. The lens is not damaged. However, the muscles that hold the lens in place must work a lot harder in order to maintain the eye's focus. This can result in blurred vision during the interchange from high blood sugar levels to low blood sugar levels and back again.

## Other Possible Signs and Symptoms of Diabetes

The following type 2 diabetes symptoms are less obvious but still important along the path to discovering your body and its potential for diabetes.

1. Changes in skin color, especially around the armpit, the neck, and the groin. The color will be darker, almost velvety.
2. Noticeably slower healing of cuts or sores.
3. Unusual skin itchiness levels. This usually occurs in the groin or vaginal area.
4. Impotency, or inability to create offspring.

# Why Is It Important to Control Diabetes?

Diabetic people who are unable to control their diabetes correctly ultimately find a wide range of complications. Look to the following to better understand the importance of ultimate health to reverse or handle diabetic symptoms.

## 1. Foot problems.

Many people who mishandle their diabetes find themselves with many foot complications, like ulcers, neuropathy, and the occasional gangrene situation. Gangrene often results in amputation.

## 2. Eye problems.

People with diabetes often find themselves with cataracts, glaucoma, and diabetic retinopathy. As a result of these eye problems, many diabetic people go blind.

## 3. Loss of hearing.

Many people who are unable to treat their diabetes properly unfortunately begin to lose their hearing very early.

## 4. Loss of mental health.

People with diabetes have a greater risk of developing both anxiety and depression, which can severely alter the way they live their lives.

## 5. Stroke.

When blood glucose levels, blood pressure, and cholesterol levels find no relief, risk of stroke elevates.

Other problems include skin complications, greater bloodstream acidity, higher inflammation, uncontrolled blood pressure, greater risk of infection, and so many more. It's incredibly important to treat the body well, eat the proper foods, and begin the exercise process to give the body much-needed relief from diabetes symptoms and complications.

# 5 Easy Steps to Reverse Diabetes Symptoms

Can you actually reverse your type 2 diabetes symptoms through lifestyle alterations? It's true that you can make changes to manage your diabetes. Having the ability to completely alter the body's construction in order to eliminate all symptoms of diabetes depends on how long you've had diabetes and the general severity of your particular disease. Furthermore, it depends on your genes.

Generally speaking, people utilize the term "diabetes reversal" when they are able to live their lives easily without medication. However, they are still meant to stay on the clean, lifestyle path to maintain their reversal. Therefore, once someone has diabetes, he must always be aware of the diabetic beast coming back to get him. (Heading back to a sedentary lifestyle, complete with extra helpings of donuts, cannot be in the cards.)

# Five Steps to Reverse Diabetes

## 1. Create a fat balance in the bloodstream.

When your body and bloodstream have too many omega-6 fatty acids, your body is at an extra-high risk of maintaining and even worsening its diabetes. Therefore, it's essential to keep your omega-3 fatty acids and your omega-6 fatty acids in a balance. Furthermore, it's best to completely avoid omega-6 seed oils. Note that nearly every restaurant utilizes seed oils; monitor the number of times you go out to eat.

## 2. Always control your insulin.

Your diabetes is often a result of insulin resistance. If you hope to rebuild your insulin sensitivity, you must limit your consumption of grains, sugars, and carbohydrates. Look to vegetables, proteins, and good fats in order to fuel a ready balance of insulin. Furthermore, monitor your blood glucose levels with the glucometer, spoken about below.

## 3. Work out.

When you exercise, you boost your bodily muscles' abilities to utilize insulin. Over a period of time, your muscles can help you achieve insulin sensitivity once more. Note that you must refine your exercise regimes. According to research, short spurts of really intense exercise work to fuel better weight loss and insulin sensitivity.

# Try the following exercise regimes:

a. Break up 30 minutes of exercise throughout the day. That means: a ten-minute walk after breakfast, lunch, and dinner. Note that you can do all your exercise in one jolt. However, if you find it difficult, breaking it up works well for many people.

b. Remember to "move around" throughout the day through cleaning, always taking the stairs, and parking a further distance from your destination. Note that these things do not count toward your overall exercise; however, they're beneficial elements to fuel you with better health.

c. Wear a pedometer and make a goal to walk 10,000 steps per day. Research shows that people who wear pedometers lose more weight than people who need to lose weight who don't wear pedometers. Make it a game for yourself.

d. Write down your exercise goals in your food log and stick to them, just as you stick to your plan of always checking your blood sugar. Consider exercise your absolute necessary aspect of your new, healthy life. For example, during your first week out, plan to exercise 15 minutes on Monday, Wednesday, Friday, and Saturday through any means necessary. When you complete that small goal, you can move forward to bigger goals.

e. Never set unattainable, out-of-reach exercise goals. You will raise your stress levels and make yourself think you will never achieve weight loss or greater health.

## 4. Lower your stress levels.

When you live a life of stress, your cortisol levels shoot up. High cortisol levels often lead to insulin problems, an improper balance of hormones, and increased risks for various serious diseases.

In order to reduce your stress levels, it's important to lower your exposure to food and environmental toxins, always get enough sleep, begin to eat properly, and work through any emotional or mental problems. If necessary, talk to a mental health professional to deal with your problems head-on.

## 5. Repair your body's intestines.

If you've been eating many grain-based carbohydrates, you probably have intestinal lining inflammation or leaky gut syndrome. This further depletes your body's intestine's "good" bacteria. Therefore, you must completely eliminate grains from your diet—at least for a little while. Furthermore, look to a probiotic in order to facilitate better intestinal healing. Find a good probiotic at your local pharmacy.

# Learning to Monitor Your Own Blood Sugar

It's essential to begin to monitor your own blood sugar to avoid highs and lows and keep your insulin levels at bay. You can further monitor which foods give you serious problems and learn to stay away from them.

## You'll Require:

## 1. A Glucometer.

A glucometer is a finger-prick machine. All diabetics utilize this machine to test their blood sugar levels.

## 2. Test strips.

These test strips must completely match the glucometer you've bought. Note that strips can be expensive.

## 3. A small journal.

When you have a small journal, you can note exactly what you've eaten and the subsequent reading you achieve on the glucometer.

## You'll Do:

Following the instructions of your specific glucometer, take blood sugar readings every single day for a week at the following times:

1. In the morning prior to your first drink or your first bite of food. Don't even drink water.
2. Prior to lunch.
3. Sixty minutes after lunch.
4. One hundred and twenty minutes after lunch.
5. One hundred and eighty minutes after lunch.

It's important not to eat anything during the hours after lunch, either. Do this every day for a week in order to yield appropriate data.

## Keep Your Food and Blood Sugar Log

It's very helpful to record your findings so you can understand your data. Therefore, it's essential that you keep a food log of every item you drink and every item you eat. Do this as you normally would for one week, trying not to "monitor" how much you eat or drink (but not going overboard, either). This way, you can truly understand how your diabetes is going to affect your overall lifestyle habits and what you need to change, immediately.

## What Should Your Blood Glucose Levels Be?

A normal fasting blood glucose level is anywhere below 83 mg/dL. Therefore, this is the reading you're going for prior to breakfast.

Your pre-lunch reading should be below 90 mg/dL.

Your post-sixty-minute reading should be below 140 mg/dL.

Your post-one hundred and twenty-minute reading should be below 120 mg/dL.

Your post one hundred and eighty-minute reading should be back to below 90 mg/dL.

Note that these are the numbers you're aiming for in your diabetes reversal. If your readings are high or at any time over the 140 mg/dL range, it's essential that you begin to alter your lifestyle habits through the five steps to diabetes reversal.

# Diabetic Living in the Kitchen: Shopping List

The basis of diabetes lies in the ways in which people take in food: what they choose and how their body chooses to handle those food choices to make energy. Naturally, people with diabetes are unable to handle large bouts of glucose without additional intake of insulin. Therefore, it's essential to understand what you're putting into your body in order to keep your blood glucose levels naturalized, balanced, and healthy.

## Watching Out for Sugars, Grains, and Omega-6 Oils

Remember that all forms of carbohydrates are eventually broken into glucose, which is essentially sugar. The body looks to glucose for energy, of course; however, too much glucose can become toxic in the body. Therefore—everything from a piece of whole wheat bread to your small helping of pasta is akin to a delicious bar of chocolate when it comes to the science of your body.

When the body takes in too much glucose, it attempts to store it as glycogen in the liver and the muscles. Unfortunately, this storage is limited. Therefore, the body begins to convert the glucose to saturated fat in the body. This is ultimately what happens to formulate insulin resistance, as well. The body doesn't know what to do with its excess glucose; therefore, the pancreas secretes even more insulin, thus eventually making the body resistant to insulin's effects. This ultimately leaves the body unable to respond to insulin appropriately, resulting, oftentimes, in diabetic symptoms.

Both grains and sugars initiate this awful response of storing saturated fats and creating a negative insulin resistance. Grains further cause gut inflammation, which can force an overall immune response and disease in the body. Sugar, on the other hand, elevates the bloodstream's levels of cortisol, which is the stress hormone that actually increases your body's desire to store belly fat, in particular. Belly fat, if you recall, can lead to further risks of metabolic syndrome.

So: how do you differentiate between all the different types of sugars? Should they all be avoided? Look at the following to better understand your sugar intake moving forward.

## 1. Sucrose.

Sucrose is made up of both glucose and fructose in a one-to-one ratio. It is known as table sugar and should be very, very strictly limited.

## 2. Glucose.

Glucose has been oft-mentioned in this book. It is found in nearly all foods—from pastas to vegetables. It must be limited but is essential in moderation.

## 3. Fructose.

Fructose is completely toxic when consumed outside of its original fruit formation. Fructose is generally found in high fructose corn syrup, which creates an inappropriate insulin response and fat storage.

## 4. Natural sugars like agave, honey, maple syrup, or molasses.

These natural sweeteners are found throughout the earth. They contain fructose and do boost insulin levels. However, they can be consumed by people with very good insulin sensitivity. Remember that moderation is always key.

## Avoiding Omega-6 Fatty Acids

Omega 6 fatty acids rear their heads in soybean oil, cottonseed oil, vegetable oil, canola oil, sunflower oil, and corn oil. These oils create inappropriate inflammation in the body and further damage the pancreas. Furthermore, they can alter the thyroid, which disrupts the intricate balance of the body's hormone levels. Hormone levels must be balanced in order to facilitate weight loss.

## Understanding the Glycemic Index

The glycemic index offers a measurement for how much a certain food raises your blood glucose levels. All foods are ranked in relation to straight-glucose or white bread. Note that foods with a high glycemic index boost your blood glucose levels more than foods with a medium or a low glycemic index.

Therefore, an appropriate diabetic lifestyle looks to choosing foods with medium or low glycemic indexes.

Carbohydrate foods that contain low glycemic index numbers include dried legumes and beans, vegetables without starch, many fruits, whole wheat bread, and bran cereal.

Note that foods that do NOT have carbs, like fats and meats, don't have a glycemic index. They don't contain any glucose!

## Note the following Low GI Foods (with 55 GI or less):

1. Steel-cut oats
2. Stone-ground whole wheat bread
3. Bulgar and quinoa
4. Fruits such as apples, pears and grapefruit
5. Non-starchy vegetables such as broccoli, cauliflower, celery

## Note the following Medium GI Foods (between 56 and 69 GI):

1. quick oats
2. whole wheat bread
3. wild or brown rice

## Note the following High GI Foods (above 70 GI):

1. white rice
2. rice pasta
3. rice cakes
4. pineapple
5. corn flakes and instant oatmeal
6. pumpkins
7. russet potatoes

The glycemic index of food gives you a rough estimate of how much your blood glucose levels will elevate after you eat. It's best to choose from the medium and low GI sections; however, it's important to note that oftentimes, foods with higher GIs have greater nutritional content. Proceed with caution and talk to a doctor if necessary.

## A Diabetic's Shopping List

It's essential to think about your grocery shopping and your pantry in a completely different light.

Begin with a complete make over. Clean out your refrigerator and your pantry. Remove all toxic foods—processed foods, saturated fat-rich foods, candy, grains, and breads.

During your next foray into the grocery store, try to shop on the outside aisles first before diving into the processed, canned food aisles. Furthermore, put some of the following things into your cart:

## Vegetables and Fruits:

Broccoli

Brussels Sprouts

Eggplant

Onion

Other Non-Starchy Vegetables

Strawberries

Blueberries

Oranges

Grapefruits

Limit Banana Intake

1%, skim, or soy milk

eggs

low fat or non-fat yogurt

cottage cheese

low-fat cheese

0 trans fat margarine

fresh meats, like poultry, meat, fish

Alternately, look to the freezer section if you want vegetables, fruits, or meats to keep longer than a few days.

## Fill your spice cabinet with the following:

Low-salt and salt-free spices
Balsamic vinegar or apple cider vinegar
Salt-free herbs
Extra virgin olive oil
Cooking spray

Fill your pantry with the following. Note to limit your sodium intake. Therefore, fresh vegetables and beans are always better for your body. However, canned products can be better on a tight budget. Further note to avoid canned fruit, if possible, as it can have higher amounts of sugar:

Canned black, kidney, or cannelloni beans
Canned vegetables of your choice

Canned salmon or tuna

Oatmeal (for days when you need higher carbohydrates)

Nuts

Whole grains like bulgur or quinoa

Flax or sunflower seeds

Note that you can continue to eat things in moderation. However, it's essential to monitor your blood sugar at all times and understand the way your body reacts to certain things. This way, you are always on guard, always noting your body's rapid changes.

# Top Natural Remedies, Herbs, and Vitamins

Many natural remedies and herbs you already have in your kitchen have healing properties that actually lower your blood sugar:

## Coffee

Some of the chemicals in coffee bring medicinal benefits against diabetes. It contains a molecule called polyphenol, which works to decrease inflammation, which ultimately leads to diabetes. Furthermore, coffee has been linked to lower your risk of developing Type 2 diabetes, Alzheimer's Cancer, and stroke.

## Green Tea

Green tea is pulsing with natural antioxidants that look to reduce the body's rampant levels of free radicals. These free radicals generally react with bad cholesterol, or LDL cholesterol, in the bloodstream to increase your risk of heart attack, atherosclerosis, and stroke. When you drink the green tea, you dramatically lower your free radical levels and work to reduce your risk of serious disease and complications from your diabetes.

## Aloe Vera

Aloe vera stems from a prickly succulent plant and has been known to bring ready healing to many-a-sunburn. However, when utilized in herbal medicines—as it has been for thousands of years—it can help improve fasting blood glucose levels. It's been shown to decrease blood lipids or fats in the blood stream. It's further been shown to assist in rapid healing of various wounds that result as diabetes complications.

Find aloe vera at many beauty and health stores.

# Cinnamon

Cinnamon spice is surely a familiar element in any vibrant household. Unfortunately, its medicinal properties are often not known. Its utilization can be traced back many thousand years. Recent research states that cinnamon can improve blood glucose levels and further decrease your chances of even getting the disease.

While just 1 gram of cinnamon taken each day can boost your insulin sensitivity and help you reverse your type 2 diabetes, up to 6 grams should be taken to reduce bad triglycerides, LDL or bad cholesterol, and overall artery cholesterol. This, in turn, lowers high blood pressure and works to decrease your risk of serious diseases, like heart disease and stroke.

Furthermore, cinnamon has been found to relieve stomachaches, de-clot the blood, rev the metabolism, and bring the body nutrients like calcium, manganese, and iron.

## Ginger

Bizarre-looking root ginger is a mainstay in Asian medicines and herbal treatments. A recent study links ginger with blood sugar control and the body's ability to accept glucose—without necessary insulin in the bloodstream. Therefore, ginger can reduce high blood sugar levels without boosting insulin levels.

Furthermore, ginger assists with nausea, pain, upper respiratory tract infections, and so much more.

## Other herbs to check out include:

1. Bilberry extract
2. Fenugreek
3. Okra
4. Bitter Melon

## Common Vitamins and Supplements

Look to the following vitamins to boost your metabolism and bring overall body healing:

## 1. Magnesium.

Diabetic people often have a reduced level of magnesium. This deficiency has been linked to influence the diabetic body's lack of control over blood glucose levels. Therefore, a boost of magnesium via a supplement or a vitamin is essential to rev your insulin sensitivity.

## 2. Vitamin B12.

As aforementioned, diabetes can cause rapid nerve damage throughout the body, resulting in inappropriate bodily communication and tingling appendages. However, if you take B12, you can dramatically reduce nerve damage.

## 3. Vitamin D.

Vitamin D, which is most-readily found in the sunshine, works to boost your insulin sensitivity, thus charging you toward diabetes reversal.

## 4. Zinc.

Zinc has been linked to insulin metabolism. In some cases, zinc supplements can further work to lower blood sugar levels.

In the next chapter, we'll discuss the 30 superfoods you can look to combat diabetes once diagnosed, or beat back against it if you're at risk.

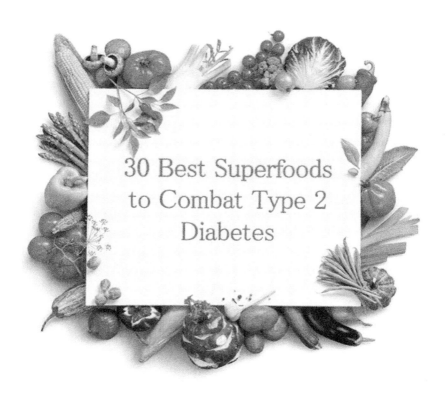

# 30 Best Superfoods to Combat Type 2 Diabetes

Stock up on the following 30 best superfoods to combat type 2 diabetes. These foods have been shown to yield maximum nutrient and vitamin intake, reduce insulin resistance, and boost overall health in diabetic individuals. Include more of these in your diet to help yourself reverse your diabetes today.

# Walnuts

A walnut is a cancer-fighting, heart-healthy nut, with several powerful antioxidants that reduce your bodily inflammation and thus reduce your body's chance of growing more insulin resistant. Furthermore, walnuts have been proven to boost metabolism of people with type 2 diabetes, resulting in better insulin levels.

# Brussels Sprouts

This delicious green vegetable is low in carbohydrates and calories, meaning they're essential to controlling your blood glucose levels. Furthermore, the fiber in Brussels sprouts binds to acids in your digestion, after steaming, which ultimately results in decreasing your bad cholesterol levels.

# Apples

According to research reported in Best Health Magazine, women who eat just a single apple per day are up to 28 percent less likely to develop diabetes down the line. This is because apples are pulsing with fiber, which makes sure your blood sugar levels don't rise or drop too quickly.

# Bok Choy

Bok choy, originally from Asian countries, is rich in antioxidants that reduce your risk of cancer and cardiovascular disease. Since type 2 diabetes puts you at a greater risk for these diseases, plan to eat more Bok choy to manage your lifestyle and keep yourself healthy.

# Avocadoes

Avocadoes are incredibly low in carbohydrates and are pulsing with healthy fats—ones that don't elevate the bad cholesterol in your system. Avocadoes also boast a ton of vitamins, including vitamin E, B, K, and potassium, along with powerful antioxidants proven to protect your eyes from cataracts, another side-effect of type 2 diabetes.

# Salmon

Salmon is one of the greatest superfoods, with a high omega-3 fatty acid and protein content. It guards against heart attacks, strokes, and cancers, and can be one of the greatest forces in your weight loss goals, since it promotes ketosis and muscle gain.

## Spinach

Spinach is incredibly rich in minerals and vitamins, as well as phytonutrients, which fight against cancer and inflammation. Spinach is very low in fat and carbs, as well, and has been proven to regulate hunger and keep you satiated.

## Cauliflower

Cauliflower, which is used in this book to create a low-carb crust for pizza, contains sulforaphane, which has been shown to reduce cancer growth. It's also rich in minerals and vitamins that boost your brain functionality and reduce inflammation.

## Scallops

Scallops, which are "fish" that don't necessarily have a fishy flavor, are rich in vitamin B12, which converts something called homocysteine into a benign chemical. Homocysteine damages your blood vessels, and thus promotes diabetic heart disease, stroke, and heart attack.

## Collard Greens

Much like Brussels sprouts or bok choy, collard greens are cruciferous vegetables, which are low in calories and carbohydrates, and are rich in vitamin C, vitamin A, and calcium. Furthermore, they're rich in fiber, which can increase your insulin sensitivity and decrease your oxidative stress.

## Olives

Olives are some of the most vibrant, nutritional items on the planet. They reduce inflammation, are incredibly low in carbohydrates, and contain hydroxytyrosol, a phytonutrient that fights cancer.

## Edamame

Edamame is a low-calorie soybean, containing a high amount of protein and calcium. The magnesium in soy beans has been shown to regulate blood sugar, while soy protein has been shown to decrease your levels of bad cholesterol, thus fighting your risk of heart attacks and stroke.

## Strawberries

Strawberries are low in calories and high in fiber, meaning that they're a sweet treat that doesn't quickly elevate your blood sugar and then allow it to fall again. Furthermore, strawberries reduce your inflammation, thus fighting cancer and insulin resistance, and promote blood flow, which leads to quicker weight loss.

# Kiwi

Kiwis have high levels of potassium, which can balance out your electrolytes and manage your blood pressure. This can help you avoid being dehydrated, which is a common issue with type 2 diabetics. Furthermore, kiwi has a very low glycemic index, meaning it won't raise your blood sugar too quickly, or allow it to fall too fast.

# Sunflower Seeds

Sunflower seeds are rich in vitamin E, which fights against free radicals and other inflammation in the body, thus fighting cancer and decreasing insulin resistance issues. It's also filled with phytosterols, which reduces your blood's bad cholesterol levels. Its high amount of magnesium also prevents migraines, while reducing the risk of stroke and heart attack.

## Asparagus

Asparagus is a natural diuretic, meaning that it contains large amounts of asparagine, which can clear out your system and reduce any excess salt—thus reducing your blood pressure. Furthermore, it contains glutathione, which fights against free radicals and inflammation. It also contains vitamin K, E, A, and C, along with fiber and folate, making it an all-around great vegetable.

## Flaxseed

Flaxseed is a low-carb food, with vitamins and minerals that improve your digestion, reduce your sugar cravings, balance your hormones, and boost weight loss. It's one of the best forms of omega-3 fatty acid on the planet, which fights inflammation and improves insulin sensitivity.

# Kale

Kale is also related to bok choy and cauliflower, and is nutritionally dense, providing more than your daily allowance of vitamin K, vitamin A, and vitamin C per day. It's surprisingly high in protein, and is loaded with antioxidants like quercetin and kaempferol, which fight oxidative damage, aging, and cancers.

# Chia Seeds

Chia seeds are an ancient food from Mexico, which reduce the signs of aging, build stronger bones, and help to fight diabetic effects. The seeds are high in fiber, meaning they won't spike your blood sugar, and they reduce inflammation, reducing your risk of heart attack and stroke.

# Broccoli

Broccoli is cousins with kale, bok choy, and cauliflower, and has been linked to decrease type 2 diabetes symptoms due to its high fiber content, high nutritional content, and low calorie count. Furthermore, the antioxidants in broccoli have proven to take years from your appearance, as it has been shown to create new collagen, your skin's main support.

# Almonds

Almonds are rich in protein, fiber, and healthy fat, which promote blood sugar stabilization and decrease cholesterol levels. Furthermore, they're rich in antioxidants, which fight cancer and decrease insulin resistance. They're also linked to decreasing your blood pressure levels.

# Ginger

Ginger is rich with gingerol, which was often used in alternative medicines throughout history, reducing flu and cold symptoms and reducing bodily inflammation. It can dramatically reduce your blood sugar levels, one study showed that subjects who ate just two grams of ginger powder per day had lower blood sugar levels, when fasted, by a full twelve percent.

# Black Beans

Black beans, like many beans, are incredibly beneficial for your colon and lower tract, reducing inflammation. They're rich in fiber, which regulates your blood sugar and fights cardiovascular disease down the line.

## Pumpkin

Pumpkins aren't just the orange orbs you carve up during October. They contain over 200 percent of your daily amount of vitamin A, protect your skin with carotenoids, and have plenty of fiber to regulate blood sugar.

## Garlic

Like ginger, garlic was often given to sick patients, as it contains medicinal, anti-inflammatory benefits. It's high in manganese, selenium, fiber, and vitamin B6, and can reduce blood pressure, thus reducing your risk of cardiovascular disease.

## Lentils

With their high fiber content, lentils have been proven to help reduce your cholesterol and stabilize your blood sugar. They're also an excellent source of vegetable protein, which aids in weight loss and revs your metabolism.

## Buckwheat

Buckwheat has a high level of rutin, which is often used to treat high blood pressure. It's also high in protein, which promotes weight loss, along with antioxidants, which reduce inflammation.

## Matcha

Matcha is an ancient form of green tea, which detoxifies your body, decreases inflammation, promotes relaxation, and stabilizes your blood sugar levels. When you drink matcha, you're ingesting the entire leaf, meaning you ingest all of the essential properties, boosting your immune system. Also, matcha tea has been shown to reduce type 2 diabetes damage in the kidneys.

## Pistachios

Pistachios provide heart health, reduce your levels of bad cholesterol, and offer tons of blood sugar-leveling fiber. They also has aphrodisiac properties, which doesn't necessarily assist with your type 2 diabetes. However, this information might improve your life.

## Cranberries

Cranberries are high in antioxidants and nutrients, offering just 25 calories per half cup. They cleanse your system, becoming an essential hack against urinary tract infections, and reduce your risk of developing cardiovascular disease down the line.

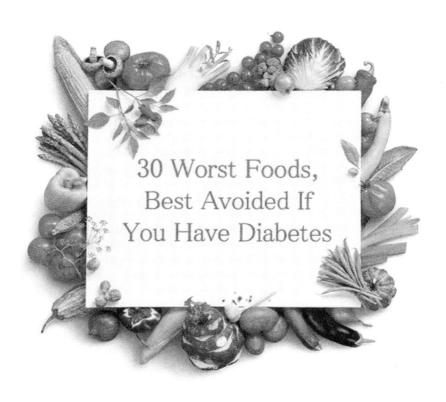

# 30 Worst Foods, Best Avoided If You Have Diabetes

The following foods are best avoided if you have type 2 diabetes, as they raise your blood sugar levels sharply, promote cardiovascular disease, and can contribute to weight gain.

# Fried Potatoes, such as tater tots or French fries

Fried potatoes change immediately to glucose in your system, which your body isn't able to use for fuel right away. Plus, when you fry your potatoes, you're adding an extra dose of grease to the mixture, which causes your cardiovascular system to work even harder to push blood to your heart. Instead of fried potatoes, try a baked, non-starchy vegetable, or sweet potatoes.

## Fruit Juices

For many, this comes as a surprise. After all, fruit juice is derived from fruit, which is the "good" kind of sugar, adding a dose of fiber-rich carbohydrates to your system. However, fruit juices contain sugar, and only sugar, and thusly force your blood sugar to spike. Plus, they're high in calories, which ultimately leads to weight gain.

## Dried Fruit

Sure, dried fruits aren't quite as bad as cookies, cakes, or pies. But they'll still spike your blood sugar as raisins and other dried fruits provide a concentrated amount of sugar, which is absorbed quickly into the bloodstream. Instead of raisins, stick to grapes.

## White Bread and White Pasta

Despite the food pyramid's assurance that white bread, and other grains, should be the "number one food" of your day, white breads and pastas turn immediately to sugar the moment your body begins to digest them. However, if you want to keep bread in your diet, stick to whole grains, which are higher in fiber and bring a more gradual rise of sugar in your bloodstream. Other options include: brown rice, quinoa, whole-wheat pasta and bread, and barley.

# Whole Milk and Other High-Fat Dairy

Whole milk is rich in saturated fat, which can make your body even more insulin resistant. Instead of drinking whole milk, opt for skim milk or 1% milk. Also, try to avoid full-fat cream cheeses and other cheeses, making sure to choose lower-fat options.

# Bacon

It's true, bacon, much like whole milk, contains a high amount of saturated fat, which boosts your body's inflammation and adds to your insulin resistance. Instead of bacon, opt for low-fat burgers, turkey burgers, and even turkey bacon! Turkey bacon crisps taste almost just the same. After a while, you won't miss this fatty favorite.

## Pretzels

When you were younger, your mother gave you pretzels, thinking they were healthier than chips, right? Unfortunately, pretzels are made from white flour, salt, and yeast, without a single lick of nutrition. Plus, immediately after consumption, your body's sugar levels spike. Instead of pretzels, try something with a bit of protein, like pistachios, almonds, or Greek yogurt.

## Soda

According to the Harvard School of Public Health, people who drink sugary soda drinks have a 26% higher chance of developing diabetes. The calories are empty, meaning they contain no nutrients your body can use. They're best avoided.

## Specialty Coffee Drinks

I'm not saying you need to eliminate coffee from your diet completely. However, drinking a bit of coffee with milk is far different than drinking Starbucks-quality, high-sugar, high-fat lattes and mochas. Each one of those drinks packs over 300 calories, depending, and can have over 60 grams of carbohydrates. Furthermore, drinks with caffeine raise your heart rate and your blood pressure, which increases inflammation, and can increase your insulin resistance.

## Preserves, Jams, and Jellies

Much like the dried fruit and fruit juices, fruit from preserves, in the form of jams and jellies, often have all the condensed sugar from their fruit-state, plus added sugar to enhance their flavor.

## Chips

Much like French fries, chips are fried, and when consumed regularly, can ultimately lead to weight gain. Furthermore, their starch content revs the sugar levels in your bloodstream immediately, and the level of LDL cholesterol (the bad kind) in chips boosts your risk of cardiovascular problems.

## Butter

As if you thought life couldn't get worse without your preserves, jams, and jellies on your toast, here's another spread you should use sparingly, if at all. Butter is high in saturated fats, which can raise your level of LDL cholesterol and also result in weight gain and cellular inflammation, leading to increased insulin resistance.

## Candy

Your sweet tooth is something you're going to have to ignore from now on. Candy, and other desserts, cause a spike in your blood sugar levels, and lead to rapid weight gain. Both of these ramp up your diabetes complications.

However, you don't have to eliminate all desserts, if you plan accordingly and keep your servings fairly small.

## Frozen Meals

In our busy lives, convenience seems key. However, many convenient meals, which you can cook in the microwave in no time at all, are actually elevating your diabetes symptoms, as they contain copious amounts of fat and sodium.

Fortunately, frozen food is coming along, making American Diabetes Association-approved meals, with less than 500 calories per serving. They recommend Smart Ones, Lean Cuisine, and Amy's Low in Sodium dishes, but also maintain that cooking your own food at home is much more beneficial, allowing you to track your healthy, fibrous carbohydrate intake, as well as your sodium.

## Milk Shakes

Milk shakes are obviously packed with calories. You already knew that. But they also contain trans fat, which is absolutely horrible for your cardiovascular system. Plus, the high carbohydrate and sugar content elevates your blood sugar levels immediately.

## Grocery Store or Fast Food Smoothies

While it's okay to make your own smoothie at home—especially one that's centered on green vegetables, rather than fruit—it's best to avoid buying smoothies at the grocery store or fast food restaurants. They look amazing, sure, with their bright colors and purported nutrition. However, many smoothies have over 200 calories and upwards of 50 carbohydrates per serving.

## White Rice

As mentioned, white breads and white pastas elevate your blood sugar immediately. But white rice, which is often regarded as "healthy" due to its relation to Asian cuisine, has a similar effect, and further contains many preservatives. Opt for brown rice or barley instead.

## Battered Fish Such as Fish and Chips

While fish is generally good for you, battered fish has tons of calories and grams of fat, with one American portion ultimately taking you over

3,000 mg of sodium per day, 100 grams of carbohydrates, and 80 grams of fat.

## High-Fructose Corn Syrup

High-fructose corn syrup, which is often used in many household favorites, such as pickle relish, salad dressings, and ketchup, is difficult to metabolize and increases your insulin resistance.

## Processed Cereals

The popular cereals we eat every morning aren't good for us, bringing us to shove upwards of 50 grams of carbohydrates per serving into our system, all without fiber. Instead of eating high-sugary cereals, try to search for ones with high levels of fiber, or even ones with added protein.

## Hot Dogs

Like bacon, hot dogs are high in saturated fats, and thus increase your body's inflammation and insulin resistance. They're also generally made up of a bunch of odds-and-ends, and are inorganic. Try turkey hot dogs, or none at all.

## Burgers

Naturally, burgers are something best avoided, unless you opt for the lower-fat variety. Burgers can raise your cholesterol levels, and thus put you at a higher risk for cardiovascular disease. Furthermore (especially if you're purchasing at a fast food or other restaurant), they're caloric bombs, often with upwards of 1,000 calories per serving.

## Processed Lunch Meat

Despite having good protein, processed lunchmeat is best resisted, as it has an incredible amount of sodium. Instead of opting for processed deli meat, opt for healthier options for lunch, like chicken salads, or veggie sandwiches.

## Muffins

Muffins are pure sugar (yes, even the ones with blueberries in them). Furthermore, they often contain trans fats, which can increase your LDL cholesterol levels. If you're not baking your muffins at home (and thus know precisely what's in them), make sure you read your nutritional labels.

## Energy Bars

While it seems easy to just grab an energy bar and run out the door, know that many of them are just as bad as most candy bars. Instead of choosing sugary bars, look for ones made of whole grains and nuts—or opt for apples, cheeses, almonds, other snacks that are filling and portable.

## Pizza

One of our favorite foods (that we don't necessarily have to give up, if we follow some better, more healthful recipes) is pulsing with carbohydrates, saturated fats, and sodium. Plus, it's a calorie bomb, and nearly impossible just to have one slice.

## Whole Eggs

Despite eggs being a "superfood," they contain a high amount of fat, ultimately doubling your risk of cardiovascular disease. However, yolk is the part of the egg that contains fat and cholesterol, meaning that you can eat egg whites since they contain all the protein. In order to replace a single egg, simply use two egg whites.

## Ketchup

America's favorite condiment, ketchup has a high amount of sugar and sodium, which gives your blood sugar a mighty spike before causing it to fall quickly. Instead of ketchup, opt for mustards, vinegars, or spices.

## Melons and Peaches

Unfortunately, while many fruits are wonderful for you, melons and peaches are higher in sugar than most, and can cause your blood sugar to spike. Instead, look to blueberries, apples, or other berries, which cause a slower rise of blood sugar.

# Chinese Food

Chinese food is not suitable to eat on a regular basis for many reasons. It's high fat, high-calorie, with tons of carbohydrates, and sodium. This can spike your blood sugar levels, and then keep your blood sugar up for a long time, which can contribute to increased inflammation. If you decide to cook Chinese food at home, make sure to never use white rice, and look to low-sodium condiments.

In the next chapter, we'll dive into the superfood recipes that will decrease your diabetes symptoms and help you lose weight.

# Diabetes-Friendly Recipes to Maximize Healing and Reversal

The key to managing your diabetes and your blood sugar lies in keeping track of your carbohydrates. As mentioned previously, carbohydrates break down into glucose in your system upon digestion. Too much glucose is seriously detrimental to your health; it may be part of the reason you currently have diabetes because it led to ultimate insulin resistance.

Therefore, the following recipes have no more than 15 grams carbohydrates. It's essential that you keep track of each serving and each carbohydrate to make sure you don't overdo your carb intake.

A Note on BMI, Calories and Carbs

The amount of carbs you should have per day generally alters based on how many calories you eat, your size, and your relative exercise level. In order to understand how many calories you should have per day, it's essential to calculate your BMI or body mass index. This is your weight-to-height ratio, created by dividing your weight (in kilos) by your height (in meters squared). If your number is lower than 18.5, you are underweight. If your BMI is between 18.5 and 24.9, you are at normal weight. If you're between 25 and 29.9, you are overweight. And if you're over 30, you're considered obese. It's important to remember that your BMI does not take into account your skeletal structure; therefore, if you're five feet tall with a medium bone structure, you might weigh a bit more than someone who is five feet tall with a small bone structure. Therefore, you need to eat a little bit more, and you are not considered overweight as a result.

If your BMI shows you're either overweight or obese, it's essential that you begin to decrease the amount of calories you eat per day. If you are a female, you should probably eat between 1,200 and 2,200 calories per day, depending on your size and your lifestyle. If you are a male, you should probably eat between 1,600 and 2,500 calories per day, depending on your activity level and other factors.

Regardless of the amount of calories you eat per day, it's essential that you limit your carb intake to about fifty percent of your total calories. You should split these calories and carbohydrates throughout your day in order to maximize your body's ability to maintain a healthy blood sugar level.

With this in mind, find the following superfood breakfasts, lunches, and dinner recipes to fuel yourself with vibrant energy and work toward a healthier lifestyle.

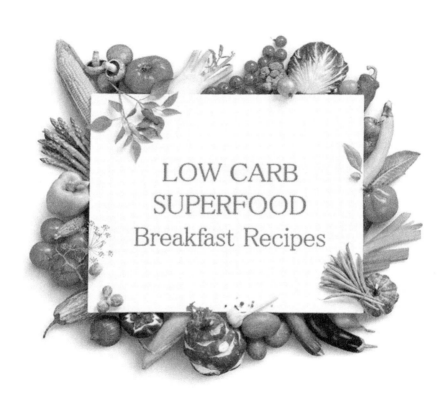

# LOW CARB SUPERFOOD Breakfast Recipes

# Green Perfection Matcha Bowl

**Recipe Makes 4 Servings.**

**Preparation Time:** 5 minutes

Nutritional Information Per Serving: 230 calories, 11 grams net carbohydrates, 4 grams protein, 18 grams fat.

**Ingredients:**

4 cups spinach, loosely-packed

¼ cup cashews, raw and soaked for 30 minutes, then drained

1 banana, frozen

2 tsp. vanilla extract

1/3 cup mint leaves

1 cups almond milk

1 tbsp. cocoa nibs

Chopped almonds, hemp seeds, cocoa nibs, puffed quinoa, etc. for toppings in the bowl

**Directions:**

Bring the listed ingredients, except for the cocoa nibs, into a blender. Blend until completely smooth. Afterwards, add the cocoa to the blender, blend for about five seconds, and then pour into four separate bowls, for serving (or just one, if you're saving the rest for later). Add the toppings of your choice, comfortable in the knowledge that they're all superfoods, and enjoy.

# Cinnamon Apple Flaxseed Waffles

**Recipe Makes 10 waffles.**

**Preparation Time:** 30 minutes

Nutritional Information Per Waffle: 169 calories, 6 grams net carbohydrates, 3 grams protein, 15 grams fat.

**Ingredients:**

1 ¼ cup almond flour

1/3 cup sweetener, low-carb, I used Swerve

½ cup flax seed meal

2 tsp. baking powder

1 tbsp. cinnamon, ground

4 eggs

1 cup almond milk

1 tsp. vanilla

1/3 cup melted butter

1 ¼ cup chopped apples

**Directions:**

First, preheat your waffle iron on medium. Grease it with a bit of butter or oil.

Next, stir together the flax seed, almond flour, sweetener, cinnamon, and the baking powder in a large bowl until well combined.

Next, add the almond milk, apples, eggs, butter, and the vanilla extract. Stir well.

Next, add three tbsp. of batter onto the waffle iron, spreading out the tablespoons so that it will evenly spread. Cook each waffle for about five minutes, or until it's golden brown. This timing will depend on your waffle iron.

Next, remove your waffles, and repeat the process until you've gotten through the batter.

Serve with no-sugar syrup, and enjoy.

# Low Carb Egg White Omelet

**Recipe Makes 1 Serving.**

**Preparation Time:** 15 minutes

Nutritional Information Per Serving: 111 calories, 1 gram net carbohydrate, 14 grams protein, 4 grams fat.

**Ingredients:**

1 tsp. olive oil

4 egg whites

1 tsp. chopped parsley

½ tsp. salt

¼ cup cooked spinach

1 tbsp. grated Parmesan

**Directions:**

First, add the olive oil to a small skillet, heating it over low heat.

To the side, whisk together the egg whites, salt, and parsley.

When the skillet is warmed, pour the eggs into the skillet. Shake the skillet back and forth over the heat, stirring at the eggs with a spatula for about a minute.

Now, place the skillet back on the heat. Add the spinach to the top of one half of the flat egg omelet. Fold the omelet at this time, making sure to cover the toppings.

Press on the omelet with your spatula to seal it. When the bottom is cooked completely, flip the omelet. Cook for an additional 30 seconds, before sliding the omelet onto a plate and topping with grated Parmesan. Serve warm, and enjoy.

# Low Carb Cinnamon "Oatmeal"

**Recipe Makes 6 Servings.**

**Preparation Time:** 15 minutes

Nutritional Information Per Serving: 372 calories, 5 grams net carbohydrates, 5 grams protein, 36 grams fat.

**Ingredients:**

¼ cup flax seed meal

1 cup pecans, crushed

3 cups coconut milk

3 ounces low-fat cream cheese

½ cup riced cauliflower

1/3 cup chia seeds

2 tsp. cinnamon

3 tbsp. low-fat, low-sodium butter

1 tsp. vanilla

½ tsp. nutmeg

¼ tsp. Allspice

10 drops liquid stevia

**Directions:**

First, measure out the flax seeds and the chia seeds, place them in a bowl together, and set them to the side.

To the side, rice the cauliflower in a food processor until ground. Set the cauliflower to the side.

Next, place the pecans in a Ziploc baggie, and then crush them. I used a rolling pin. Place the pecans in a skillet, and heat them over low heat.

Next, heat the coconut milk in a saucepan over medium heat. After it's warm, add the cauliflower to the milk, increase the heat to medium-high, and cook until the cauliflower and milk begin to boil.

Turn down the heat to medium-low. Add all the seasonings listed above, including the stevia. Stir well between each addition.

Add the chia seeds, and the flax seed to the saucepan, and stir well. This will thicken the "oatmeal."

Next, measure out the low-fat butter and cream cheese. Add these, along with the pecans, to the hot mixture, and stir well, until melted. Serve warm, and enjoy.

# Healthy Morning Muffins

**Recipe Makes 8 muffins.**

**Preparation Time:** 30 minutes

Nutritional Information Per Serving: 80 calories, 4 grams net carbohydrates, 4 grams protein, 5 grams fat.

**Ingredients:**

1 ¼ cup almond flour

1 tsp. baking powder

1 egg

1 shot of brewed coffee

1/3 cup almond milk

1/3 cup Greek yogurt, plain

2 tsp. vanilla

1 tbsp. maple syrup

**Directions:**

First, preheat the oven to 355 degrees Fahrenheit.

Stir together the almond flour, baking powder, egg, coffee, almond milk, Greek yogurt, vanilla, and the maple syrup until smooth. Add the batter to the muffin tins, filling them approximately ¾ of the way full. Bake for 20 minutes, and then remove from the oven.

Allow them to cool, and enjoy. They'll keep for about four days at room temperature, and much longer in the fridge.

# British Blueberry Popovers with Fruit Salad Topping

**Recipe Makes 8 Servings.**

**Preparation Time:** 45 minutes

Nutritional Information Per Serving: 143 calories, 8 grams net carbohydrates, 3 grams protein, 10 grams fat.

**Ingredients:**

1 cup almond flour

1 tsp. sugar

½ tsp. salt

2 eggs

1 cup almond milk

¾ cup blueberries

**Berry topping:**

1 cup blueberries

1 cup raspberries

2 tsp. maple syrup

1 cup strawberries

**Directions:**

First, preheat the oven to 425 degrees Fahrenheit.

Stir together the salt and the almond flour. Add the sugar, and stir well, creating a hole in the center of the mixture. Break the eggs into the center of this hole, along with the almond milk. Once added, beat the mixture together with a fork.

Once the batter is smooth, divide the batter into eight of the muffin tins. Add blueberries to the batter in each muffin tin. Add water to the empty muffin tins, filling them half full.

Next, bake the popovers for 30 minutes, until they're golden brown and crispy.

As the popovers bake, puree the raspberries, strawberries, and blueberries together. Add the maple syrup and stir well. Remove the popovers from the muffin tin after cooling, and top them with the berry salad.

# Low Carb Coconut Flour Garlic Bagels

**Recipe Makes 6 Servings.**

**Preparation Time:** 20 minutes

Nutritional Information Per Serving: 167 calories, 2 grams net carbohydrates, 6 grams protein, 14 grams fat.

**Ingredients:**

1/3 cup low-sodium, low-fat butter or margarine

6 eggs

½ cup coconut flour, sifted

½ tsp. salt

½ tsp. baking powder

2 tsp. garlic powder

**Directions:**

Preheat the oven to 400 degrees Fahrenheit.

First, stir together the eggs, salt, butter, and the garlic powder until well combined.

To the side, stir together the coconut flour with the baking powder. Add the coconut flour to the egg mixture, and beat well until the mixture contains no lumps.

Spoon the mixture into a donut pan. Cook the bagels for 15 minutes, and then allow them to cool.

# Kale and Sweet Potato Hash

**Recipe Makes 4 Servings.**

**Preparation Time:** 20 minutes.

Nutritional Information Per Serving: 143 calories, 14.9 grams net carbohydrates, 1 gram protein, 7 grams fat.

**Ingredients:**

1 tsp. cumin, ground

2 tbsp. olive oil

1 red onion

1 1/2 cups sweet potatoes, diced

½ tsp. garlic powder

½ tsp. paprika

1 tsp. pepper

1 bunch kale, sliced

**Directions:**

First, heat a skillet over medium heat. Add the onion and the olive oil, sautéing the onion for about five minutes.

Add the sweet potato to the skillet at this time, cooking for nine minutes, stirring often.

Next, add the spices to the sweet potato and onion, including the cumin, paprika, coriander, and pepper. Stir well to coat.

Add the kale at this time, and cook for two minutes, or until it's wilted.

Serve the kale and sweet potatoes warm, and enjoy.

# Quinoa and Pomegranate Morning Porridge

**Recipe makes 4 Servings.**

**Preparation Time:** 10 minutes

Nutritional Information Per Serving: 141 calories, 12 grams net carbohydrates, 2 grams protein, 9 grams fat.

**Ingredients:**

2 plums, sliced into bite-sized pieces

1/2 cup quinoa flakes

2 tsp. cinnamon

1/2 cups almond milk

pulp from a ¼ pomegranate, taken apart

¼ cup coconut flakes

**Directions:**

Add the quinoa and the almond milk to a saucepan, and heat on medium heat for four minutes, stirring occasionally. The mixture should be smooth.

Add the cinnamon and the coconut at this time, and stir.

Add the plums and the pomegranate, stir well, and serve warm.

# Spinach Egg White Quiche

**Recipe Makes 6 Servings.**

**Preparation Time:** 1 hour and 25 minutes

Nutritional Information Per Serving: 190 calories, 4 grams net carbohydrates, 9 grams protein, 15 grams fat.

**Ingredients:**

1 tbsp. olive oil

1 cup sliced squash, yellow

2 cups sliced zucchini

1 sliced green pepper

1 tbsp. chopped thyme

3 minced garlic cloves

8 large egg whites

1 cup almond milk

½ cup shredded cheese, low-sodium

½ tsp. black pepper

1 tbsp. grated Parmesan cheese

**Directions:**

Begin by placing a skillet on the stovetop over medium-high heat. Add the olive oil, along with the zucchini and squash, garlic, green pepper, and thyme. Stir often, cooking the vegetables for about eight minutes. After they're tender, add the vegetables to a bowl and set the bowl to the side.

Next, preheat your oven to 350 degrees Fahrenheit.

Next, in a separate bowl, stir together the egg whites, milk, and pepper until well-combined.

Add the vegetables to the bottom of a pie pan. Add the shredded cheese over the vegetables, and then top the vegetables and cheese with the egg. Sprinkle the parmesan over the eggs.

Next, bake the quiche for 45 minutes, or until it's set. Cool the quiche for 10 minutes, and then slice and serve.

# Breakfast Smoothie - Almond Milk and Flax Seed Smoothie

**Recipe Makes 1 Serving.**

**Nutritional Breakdown Per Serving:** 360 calories, 15 grams carbohydrates, 8 grams protein, 30 grams fat.

**Ingredients:**

½ cup Almond Breeze milk

1 tbsp. flax oil

¼ cup soaked almonds

½ cup sliced strawberries

2 tbsp. flax seeds

3 ice cubes

3 ounces filtered water

**Directions:**

Bring all of the above ingredients together in a blender and blend them thoroughly to your desired consistency. Enjoy.

# Breakfast Smoothie - Satisfying Rice-Based Protein Shake

**Recipe makes 1 Serving.**

Nutritional Breakdown Per Serving: 493 calories, 18 grams carbohydrates, 32 grams protein, 30 grams fat.

**Ingredients:**

1 tbsp. flax oil

2 scoops Vegan Rice Protein Powder

3 ice cubes

2 tbsp. flaxseeds

½ cup blueberries

¼ cup soaked almonds

6 ounces water

**Directions:**

Bring the above ingredients together in a blender and blend them until completely smooth. Enjoy!

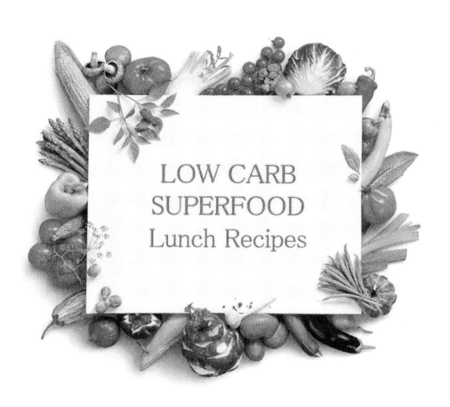

# LOW CARB SUPERFOOD Lunch Recipes

# Flaxseed Bread for Healthy, Superfood Sandwiches

**Recipe Makes 6 Servings.**

**Preparation Time:** 45 minutes

Nutritional Information Per Serving: 372 calories, 1 gram net carbohydrate, 12 grams protein, 28 grams fat.

**Ingredients:**

5 egg whites

2 ¼ cups flax seed, ground

5 ½ tbsp. coconut oil

3 egg yolks

½ cup water

½ tsp. salt

2 ½ tbsp. apple cider vinegar

## Optional Toppings for 1 Sandwich:

1 ounce smoked salmon

1 tbsp. capers

½ diced red onion

### Directions:

First, preheat the oven to 350 degrees Fahrenheit.

Next, add the egg whites to a medium-sized bowl, and whisk them until they're stiff.

To the side, blend together the oil, salt, baking powder, and flax seed until well combined.

Next, add the water, apple cinder vinegar, and egg yolks to the flax seed mixture. Stir well.

Fold the egg whites into the flax seed mixture, doing this gently until combined.

Pour the mixture into a bread pan, and bake the bread for 30 minutes.

The bread should be golden and firm. Serve with toppings of your choice.

# Avocado and Caprese Salad

**Recipe Makes 4 Servings.**

**Preparation Time:** 10 minutes

Nutritional Information Per Serving: 382 calories, 9 grams net carbohydrates, 34 grams protein, 21 grams fat.

**Ingredients:**

½ cup balsamic vinegar

1 tbsp. maple syrup

2 boneless and skinless chicken breasts, sliced

1 tbsp. olive oil

7 cups chopped lettuce, romaine

1 cup halved cherry tomatoes

1 halved and diced avocado

1/3 cup basil leaves, chopped

4 ounces fresh mozzarella, divided

**Directions:**

First, add the maple syrup and the balsamic vinegar to a small saucepan. Heat over medium, bringing it to a boil. Reduce the mixture by half. This should take about five minutes. Afterwards, set the saucepan to the side, and allow it to cool.

Next, heat the olive oil in a skillet on the stovetop, over medium heat.

Place the chicken in the skillet, and cook, flipping at least once, until you've cooked it all the way through. This should take about 8 minutes in total.

Next, make the salad by placing the lettuce in the bottom of a bowl, topping the lettuce with chicken, following that up with tomatoes, mozzarella, basil, and avocado. Add the reduction over the salad, and toss it gently. Serve the salad, and enjoy.

# Tuna and Avocado Salad

**Recipe Makes 4 Servings.**

**Preparation Time:** 10 minutes

Nutritional Information Per Serving: 210 calories, 11 grams net carbohydrates, 14 grams protein, 16 grams fat.

**Ingredients:**

10 ounces of tuna, drained from the can

3 minced garlic cloves

1 large avocado, cubed

2 tsp. spicy brown mustard

1 celery stalk, chopped

3 tbsp. minced red onion

3 tbsp. mayonnaise

1 tsp. pepper

**Directions:**

First, stir together the tuna, garlic cloves, avocado, mustard, celery, red onion, mayonnaise, and pepper in a large bowl.

Stir until the ingredients are well combined, and then serve between two whole grain pieces of bread, or overtop some leafy greens.

# Veggie Spaghetti Squash

**Recipe Makes 6 Servings.**

**Preparation Time:** 50 minutes

Nutritional Information Per Serving: 180 calories, 13 grams net carbohydrates, 6 grams protein, 9 grams fat.

**Ingredients:**

1 bunch of kale

1 spaghetti squash

4 minced garlic cloves

1 tbsp. olive oil

1 cup chickpeas from a can

½ tsp. chili powder

1 cup toasted hazelnuts

1 tbsp. grated Parmesan

**Directions:**

First, preheat the oven to 400 degrees Fahrenheit.

Next, slice the spaghetti squash in half, lengthwise, and remove all of the seeds. Place the two halves facedown on a baking sheet, and cook in the oven for 45 minutes.

While the squash bakes, wash the kale and chop it. Add the olive oil to a skillet, and then add the chili powder and the garlic to the olive oil.

Cook the garlic for two minutes. At this time, add the kale to the skillet and cook for an additional three minutes, or until the kale turns bright green.

Next, add the chickpeas to the skillet. Cook for three minutes more.

At this time, remove the squash from the oven. Use a fork to scrape out the bottom of each of the spaghetti squash halves, which ultimately forms "spaghetti-like" strands. Place the fake spaghetti into a large bowl, and toss it with the chickpea and kale.

Serve the spaghetti squash with a topping of hazelnuts and Parmesan cheese, and enjoy.

# Chickpea and Salmon Salad

**Recipe Makes 6 Servings.**

**Preparation Time:** 1 hour and 15 minutes

Nutritional Information Per Serving: 193 calories, 14 grams net carbohydrates, 13 grams protein, 7 grams fat.

**Ingredients:**

15 ounces of canned chickpeas, drained and rinsed

6 chopped stalks of celery

2 green peppers, sliced

4 minced shallots

3 minced garlic cloves

1 sliced cucumber

1 halved pint of cherry tomatoes

¼ cup olive oil

Juice from one lemon

Zest from one lemon

1 tsp. dried dill

½ tsp. smoked paprika

½ tsp. cumin

1 tsp. crushed red pepper flakes

3 six-ounce fillets of salmon, pre-cooked, and then diced

**Directions:**

Prepare your vegetables, slicing and dicing, and then add them to a large bowl. Add the chickpeas to the bowl, and then toss the chickpeas with the olive oil, lemon zest, lemon juice, dill, and spices.

Afterwards, add the chopped salmon to the bowl, and toss to combine. Allow the salad to sit in the refrigerator for about one hour, and then taste the salad and adjust the seasoning if needed.

Serve the salmon salad cold, and enjoy. This will keep in your refrigerator, covered, for about four days.

# Low Carb Mexican Soup in the Slow Cooker

**Recipe Makes 6 Servings.**

**Preparation Time:** 8 hours and 10 minutes

Nutritional Information Per Serving: 306 calories, 6 grams net carbohydrates, 40 grams protein, 11 grams fat.

**Ingredients:**

1 ¾ pound chicken, boneless and skinless

1 diced jalapeno

1 diced green pepper

1 diced onion

2 ½ cups chicken stock

1 tbsp. cumin

15 ounces tomatoes, diced

3 minced garlic cloves

1 tsp. paprika

½ tbsp. chili powder

1 tsp. pepper

3 tbsp. chopped cilantro

1 sliced avocado for topping

**Directions:**

First, place the chicken at the bottom of the crockpot.

Over the chicken, add the prepared vegetables, along with the diced tomatoes and the chicken stock.

Add the spices, and cover the slow cooker. Cook on low heat for eight hours, or on high heat for four hours. Afterwards, use two forks to shred up the chicken, and stir well.

Add the cilantro and the avocado to the top, and enjoy.

# Turkey Bacon Broccoli Salad

**Recipe Makes 4 Servings.**

**Preparation Time:** 20 minutes

Nutritional Information Per Serving: 176 calories, 11 grams net carbohydrates, 18 grams protein, 3 grams fat.

**Ingredients:**

2 ¼ pounds broccoli, chopped into bite-sized pieces

½ pound turkey bacon, pre-cooked

1 cup low-sodium mayonnaise

2 tbsp. white vinegar

4 sliced green onions

1 tsp. sesame oil

3 tbsp. Swerve

**Directions:**

First, crumble the pre-cooked turkey bacon, and slice and dice the broccoli.

Mix together the white vinegar, sesame oil, Swerve, mayonnaise and the green onions.

Assemble the salad by placing the broccoli in the bottom of a bowl, adding the turkey bacon, and then pouring the dressing over the top. Toss the salad well, and serve the salad cold.

# Black Bean and Chicken Soup

**Recipe Makes 8 Servings.**

**Preparation Time:** 35 minutes

Nutritional Information Per Serving: 147 calories, 14 grams net carbohydrates, 2 grams fat, 13 grams protein.

**Ingredients:**

2 diced chicken breasts, skinless and boneless

1 tbsp. tomato paste

1 cup chicken broth, low sodium

10 ounces black beans, drained

½ tsp. chili powder

½ tsp. onion powder

½ tsp. garlic powder

¼ tsp. cayenne powder

**Directions:**

Cook the chicken in a skillet on medium-high heat, flipping once. This should take about 10 minutes. Remove the chicken from the skillet and dice.

Next, stir together the chicken and the remaining ingredients in a large saucepan.

Simmer the soup together for about 20 minutes, stirring occasionally.

Serve warm, and enjoy.

# Flaxseed Tortilla Tacos

**Recipe Makes 6 Servings.**

**Preparation Time:** 30 minutes

Nutritional Information Per Tortilla: 147 calories, 1 gram net carbohydrate, 8 grams protein, 9 grams fat.

**Ingredients:**

6 eggs

¾ cup flaxseeds

½ tbsp. olive oil

**Stuffing Ingredients:**

½ cup black beans, drained

1 sliced avocado

1 pound pre-cooked chicken, diced

**Directions:**

First, make your tortillas. Grind the flaxseeds in your blender until the flaxseeds form a meal.

Add the eggs to the flaxseed mixture, and continue to blend the mixture until it's well combined.

Next, allow the mixture to set for about five minutes. The mixture will begin to thicken.

Heat the skillet to medium, and drop the olive oil onto it, tilting the pan to coat.

Add about a sixth of the flaxseed mixture to the skillet, using a spatula to spread it. Allow it to cook for about two minutes, or until the edges begin to separate. Flip over the tortilla at this time.

Next, brown the tortilla on the other side for about 30 seconds. Remove the tortilla from the pan, and then continue making tortillas with the remaining ingredients.

Once the tortillas are ready, you can fill them with any ingredients you like. Personally, I opted for chicken, avocado, and black beans—but you can choose anything.

# Superfood Pumpkin Soup

**Recipe Makes 3 Servings.**

**Preparation Time:** 25 minutes

Nutritional Information Per Serving: 239 calories, 8 grams net carbohydrates, 2 grams protein, 21 grams fat.

**Ingredients:**

1 cup pumpkin puree

3 tbsp. margarine or low-sodium, low-fat butter

1 ½ cups vegetable stock, low-sodium

½ tsp. minced ginger

½ tsp. cinnamon

1 tsp. pepper

½ diced onion

3 minced garlic cloves

½ tsp. nutmeg

½ tsp. coriander

1 bay leaf

½ cup coconut cream

**Directions:**

First, add the margarine or butter to a large saucepan. Heat over medium-low, allowing it to melt completely.

Next, add the onion, ginger, and garlic to the saucepan. Stir well, and allow it to sauté for three minutes. The onions should begin to be clear.

Once the onions are clear, add the remaining spices to the saucepan. Allow it to cook for an additional three minutes.

Measure out pumpkin puree and add it to the saucepan. Stir well.

After it's mixed, add the vegetable broth to the mixture, stirring until well combined.

Bring the soup to a boil. Afterwards, turn the heat to low, and allow the soup to simmer for 20 minutes.

Afterwards, utilize a blender or an immersion blender to blend the soup well. When the soup is well blended, add the coconut cream to the soup and stir well.

Serve the soup warm, and enjoy.

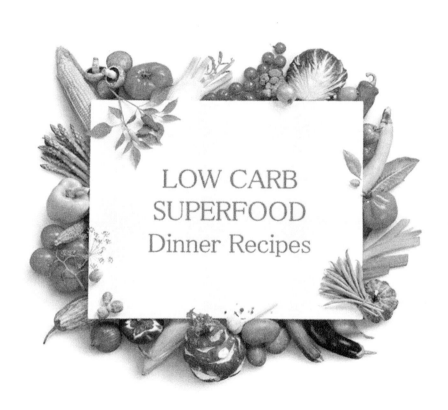

# LOW CARB SUPERFOOD Dinner Recipes

# Curried Chicken and Vegetables

**Recipe Makes 6 Servings.**

Nutritional Breakdown Per Serving: 282 calories, 18 grams carbohydrates, 18 grams protein, 15 grams fat.

**Ingredients:**

2 6-ounce chicken breasts

2 tbsp. sesame oil

1 diced onion

1 tbsp. mustard seeds

1 tbsp. curry powder

3 minced garlic cloves

1 diced carrot

2 ½ cups chopped cauliflower

1 chopped apple

1 chopped green pepper

1 cup coconut milk

1 cup frozen peas

**Directions:**

Begin by pouring the sesame oil into a large skillet and heating it over medium.

Next, add the mustard seeds. Stir the seeds for fifteen seconds, making sure they don't burn. Next, add the onions and the garlic. Sauté the mixture for a full six minutes.

Next, position the curry and the cayenne in the skillet and stir well. Add the chicken breasts to the skillet and sear it on all of its sides.

Next, pour in the coconut milk and the apple. Simmer the mixture for about twenty minutes on low. The chicken should be completely cooked.

After twenty minutes, add the frozen peas and simmer for an additional three minutes.

# Pesky Pesto Chicken with Walnuts

**Recipe Makes 4 Servings.**

Nutritional Breakdown Per Serving: 160 calories, 1 gram carbohydrate, 9 grams protein, 14 grams fat.

**Ingredients:**

1/3 pound boneless and skinless chicken

3 tbsp. extra virgin olive oil

½ tsp. sea salt

1/3 cup walnuts

1 ¾ cup fresh basil leaves

3 minced garlic cloves

**Directions:**

Begin by slicing up the chicken to create long, thin strips. Next, toss the chicken with the salt. Pour just one of the tbsp. of olive oil into a skillet and allow the chicken to griddle over medium. When the chicken is completely cooked, set it to the side.

Next, place the walnuts in a food processor and grind them until they're fine. Position the garlic, basil, and the salt in the food processor and begin the grinding process. As it grinds, add the remaining olive oil into the processor.

Next, toss the chicken strips with the created pesto, and serve.

# Chicken Shawarma with a Lemon and Basil Glaze

**Recipe Makes 4 Servings.**

**Preparation Time:** 40 minutes

Nutritional Information Per Serving: 453 calories, 2 grams net carbohydrates, 33 grams protein, 34 grams fat.

**Chicken Ingredients:**

1 pound chicken breasts, sliced into strips

3 tbsp. lemon juice

1 ½ tbsp. olive oil

1 tsp. curry powder

4 minced garlic cloves

¼ tsp. ground coriander

**Vinaigrette Ingredients:**

2 minced garlic cloves

2 handfuls basil leaves, chopped

2 tbsp. lemon juice

6 tbsp. olive oil

**Salad Bowl Ingredients**

7 cups mixed greens

2 handfuls basil leaves, chopped

1 sliced avocado

¾ cup halved cherry tomatoes

**Directions:**

First, stir together the lemon juice, garlic, curry powder, olive oil, coriander, and cumin in a small bowl. Pour this mixture into a Ziploc bag, and add the chicken. Place the chicken in the refrigerator for 30 minutes to marinate.

Next, heat the skillet over medium-high heat. Add the chicken to the skillet, cooking until it's golden brown. This should take about eight minutes.

As the chicken cooks, make the vinaigrette by blending together the lemon juice, garlic, and the basil in a food processor. As the motor continues, pour the oil into the food processor slowly. Blend well, and then set the mixture to the side.

Next, add the salad bowl ingredients to a large bowl, along with the chicken. Drizzle the dressing over the salad, toss, and serve.

# Garlic Salmon with Tomatoes

**Recipe Makes 4 Servings.**

**Preparation Time:** 15 minutes

Nutritional Information Per Serving: 324 calories, 5 grams net carbohydrates, 35 grams protein, 18 grams fat.

**Ingredients:**

4 salmon fillets, six ounces each

2 tbsp. olive oil

9 sprigs of thyme, fresh

4 halved tomatoes

½ tsp. paprika

5 minced garlic cloves

**Directions:**

First, heat your broiler.

Place the tomatoes and the salmon in a roasting pan, with the cut-side up for the tomatoes.

Drizzle the olive oil over the tomatoes and the salmon, and then season them with thyme and paprika. Add the garlic cloves.

Next, broil the salmon and tomatoes until the salmon is cooked through and the tomatoes are tender. This should take about 10 minutes.

Serve warm, and enjoy.

# Asian Salmon Coated with Black Bean Sauce

**Recipe Makes 4 Servings.**

**Preparation Time:** 35 minutes

Nutritional Information Per Serving: 497 calories, 8 grams net carbohydrates, 36 grams protein, 36 grams fat.

**Ingredients:**

2 tbsp. low-sodium soy sauce

2 tsp. cornstarch

½ cup olive oil

1 ½ cups low-sodium chicken broth

3 minced garlic cloves

4 salmon fillets, six ounces each

2 tbsp. black bean sauce

2 tsp. white wine vinegar

1/3 cup grated radishes

½ cup sliced scallions

¼ cup sliced carrots

**Directions:**

First, stir together the soy sauce and half of the olive oil in a large bowl.

To the side, stir together the cornstarch and the chicken broth in a small bowl. Set both of these bowls to the side.

Next, slice the skins in each salmon, cutting halfway into the fillet. Place the salmon fillets in a shallow baking dish, and add the soy sauce and olive oil into the dish. Refrigerate the salmon, with the soy sauce marinade, for 20 minutes.

While the salmon marinates, heat the other half of the olive oil in a saucepan over medium heat. Add the garlic, and the black bean sauce to the mixture, and stir, cooking, for two minutes. The garlic should be a golden color.

Preheat the broiler at this time.

Next, add the cornstarch, chicken broth, and vinegar to the saucepan. Cook the mixture on high, bring it to a boil, and then reduce the heat to medium to bring it to a simmer. Simmer for 10 minutes, then remove it from the heat. Keep it warm.

Next, remove the salmon from the oil mixture, pour the mixture out, and place the salmon bake in the baking dish. Broil the salmon for four minutes on each side.

Remove the salmon from the oven, and serve the salmon coated in the created sauce. Serve warm, and enjoy.

# Low Carb, Easy Scallops with Vegetable Stew

**Recipe Makes 3 Servings.**

**Preparation Time:** 30 minutes

Nutritional Information Per Serving: 200 calories, 14 grams net carbohydrates, 26 grams protein, 1.5 grams fat.

**Ingredients:**

15 ounces scallops

1 diced green pepper

2 diced tomatoes

3 minced garlic cloves

2 diced onions

½ diced eggplant

½ cup water

1 tsp. grape seed oil

**Directions:**

First, prepare a vegetable stew by tossing the green pepper, tomatoes, onions, garlic, and eggplant into a medium-sized saucepan, adding the water, and allowing it to heat until the vegetables are soft. This should take about 20 minutes.

Next, add grape seed oil to a skillet. Add scallops to the skillet, and allow the scallops to sear. Flip after each side is seared. This will take less than a few minutes.

If desired, reheat the vegetable stew. Add the scallops over the vegetable stew, and enjoy.

# Cauliflower Pizza Crust with Vegan Toppings

**Recipe Makes 2 Servings.**

**Preparation Time:** 1 hour

Nutritional Information Per Serving: 298 calories, 14 grams net carbohydrates, 20 grams protein, 7 grams fat.

**Ingredients:**

1 head of cabbage

1 tbsp. coconut flour

2 eggs

3 tbsp. nutritional yeast

1 tsp. dried oregano

2 minced garlic cloves

½ tsp. oregano, dried

½ tsp. black pepper

**Toppings:**

1 diced onion

1 cup spinach

½ cup basil pesto

½ cup broccoli florets, chopped

1 diced red pepper

**Directions:**

First, make the pizza crust.

Preheat the oven to 450 degrees Fahrenheit.

Chop the cauliflower into small pieces, and then add the cauliflower to a blender. Blend the cauliflower until it's pureed, although it doesn't have to be perfect.

Next, place the cauliflower in a saucepan, and steam it for about five minutes. It should be soft.

Next, add the cauliflower back to the blender and puree until completely smooth.

Add the cauliflower to a cheesecloth or a bunch of paper towels, and squeeze it over a large bowl to get all the water out. Allow it to sit for another five minutes before squeezing again.

Next, toss out the water from the cauliflower.

Stir the cauliflower with the coconut flour, eggs, nutritional yeast, spices,
and garlic cloves, either hand mixing or using a large wooden spoon.

Spread the cauliflower crust on a piece of parchment paper in a circular, pizza-crust fashion, making sure to leave it about ½ an inch thick.

Bake the pizza crust for 20 minutes. The top should be golden. Remove the pizza crust from the oven, and top it with the ingredients—and any others of your choice. Bake for another 12 minutes at 400 degrees Fahrenheit.

Serve the pizza warm, and enjoy.

# Asian Asparagus and Turkey

**Recipe Makes 4 Servings.**

**Preparation Time:** 20 minutes

Nutritional Information Per Serving: 219 calories, 9 grams net carbohydrates, 23 grams protein, 9 grams fat.

**Ingredients:**

1/3 cup chicken broth

2 tsp. cornstarch

1 pound turkey breast, sliced into strips

1 tsp. soy sauce

2 tbsp. lemon juice

2 minced garlic cloves

2 tbsp. olive oil

1 ¼ pound asparagus, trimmed, sliced into bite-sized pieces

**Directions:**

First, stir together the chicken broth, lemon, cornstarch, and soy sauce in a medium-sized bowl. Set the mixture to the side.

Next, add the turkey, 1 tbsp. of the oil, and the garlic to a skillet or wok. Stir fry the turkey until the meat isn't pink. Next, remove the turkey from the heat, but make sure to keep it warm.

Add the asparagus to the skillet, and cook until they're crispy. Add the broth mixture to the skillet, and cook for one minute, until it's thick.

Return the turkey to the skillet, and cook until heated. Serve the asparagus turkey dinner warm, and enjoy.

# Walnut Dinner Salad with Feta and Cranberries

**Recipe Makes 4 Servings.**
**Preparation Time:** 10 minutes

Nutritional Information Per Serving: 467 calories, 8 grams net carbohydrates, 13 grams protein, 35 grams fat.

**Ingredients:**

2 ½ cups mixed baby greens,

5 ounces feta cheese, crumbed

¾ cup dried cranberries

½ tbsp. honey

2 tbsp. balsamic vinegar

1 cup toasted walnut pieces

½ tsp. pepper

1 tsp. Dijon mustard

1/3 cup olive oil

**Directions:**

First, toss together the greens, cheese, cranberries, and walnuts in a large salad bowl.

Next, stir together the honey, oil vinegar, pepper, and mustard.

Pour the mixture over the salad, and toss it to coat. Serve the salad immediately, and enjoy.

# Pistachio and Kale Pesto with Halibut

**Recipe Makes 4 Servings.**

**Preparation Time:** 20 minutes

Nutritional Information Per Serving: 553 calories, 3 grams net carbohydrates, 65 grams protein, 28 grams fat.

**Pesto Ingredients:**

4 packed cups of kale

5 peeled cloves of garlic

2 cups basil, fresh

zest from a lemon

juice from a lemon

1 cup roasted pistachios, shelled

½ cup olive oil

½ cup Parmesan cheese, grated

**Halibut Ingredients:**

4 slices of lemons

¾ cups pesto

4 four-ounce halibut fillets

1 tbsp. olive oil

**Directions:**

First, make the pesto, which will yield far more than you require for the halibut (but it's delicious on salads later).

Combine the zest, garlic cloves, and the pistachios in a food processor. Pulse until chopped. Then, add the lemon juice, basil, and kale. Blend well. Next, add the olive oil slowly, through the top, blending ad scraping down the sides every so often, to incorporate all pieces.

Next, transfer the pesto to a bowl, and add the Parmesan cheese. Stir well. Reserve three-quarters of a cup to the side, and freeze the rest.

Next, add olive oil to a skillet, and heat the skillet over medium-high. Place the halibut on the skillet, squeezing a bit of lemon juice over each halibut fillet.

Cook the fillets for about four minutes, then flip them. The fish should be cooked all the way through and flaky.

Remove the halibut from the heat, and serve with pesto over it.

# Edamame Veggie Burger

**Recipe Makes 8 Burgers.**

**Preparation Time:** 1 hour and 30 minutes

Nutritional Information Per Serving: 123 calories, 10 grams net carbohydrates, 9 grams protein, 4 grams fat.

**Ingredients:**

1/3 cup millet

1/3 cup water, cold

½ tsp. salt

1 radish, large

1 carrot

2 minced garlic cloves

2 tbsp. peeled and grated ginger

2 tbsp. white rice vinegar

¼ tsp. Asian chili paste

2 egg whites, beaten

1 pound peeled edamame

1 cup panko breadcrumbs

**Directions:**

First, add the millet to a saucepan, adding a lid. Heat over medium-high, shaking occasionally, until the seeds begin to make a popping sound. Allow the seeds to toast for about two minutes.

Next, add the water and the salt to the saucepan. Bring the water to a boil at high heat. Place the lid over the saucepan, and then lower the heat to the lowest setting. Simmer the water for 20 minutes. Afterwards, remove the saucepan from the heat, and set it to the side for 10 minutes. At this time, fluff the millet with a fork. Add the millet to a large bowl to the side.

Next, grate the radish and the carrot, adding it to the millet bowl. Add the garlic, ginger, rice vinegar, and the chili paste, stirring well.

Next, bring a large pot of water to a boil. Add the edamame to the water, cover it, and bring the water back to a boil. Cook the edamame until it's soft. This should take about five minutes. Drain the edamame and add it to the millet bowl. Stir and set the mixture to the side to allow the edamame to cool.

After it cools, add the mixture to a food processor, and puree the mixture into a smooth paste. Return the mixture to a bowl, and add the panko and the egg whites. Stir until well combined.

Next, form the edamame mixture into patties, and place them on a baking sheet covered with parchment paper. Refrigerate them until they're set.

Next, place the oven rack about four inches away from the broiler. Preheat the broiler, and place the baking sheet beneath the broiler. Broil for about three minutes. Then, remove the patties, flip them, and broil for an additional three minutes.

Serve warm, with low-carb bread or naan, and enjoy.

# Skillet with Apples, Chicken, Sweet Potatoes, and Brussels Sprouts

**Recipe Makes 4 Servings.**

**Preparation Time:** 50 minutes

Nutritional Information Per Serving: 358 calories, 14 grams carbohydrates, 38 grams protein, 12 grams fat.

**Ingredients:**

1 tbsp. olive oil

3 cups quartered Brussels sprouts

1 pound chicken breasts, boneless and skinless, chopped into bite-sized pieces

1 sweet potato, peeled and sliced into cubes

1 diced onion

2 peeled, cored, and cut apples

1 tsp. cinnamon

½ tsp. dried thyme

5 minced garlic cloves

1 cup chicken broth

**Directions:**

Add olive oil to a large skillet and heat it over medium-high, until it's simmering. Add the chicken to the skillet, and cook for about five minutes. Transfer the chicken to a separate plate.

Next, add the Brussels sprouts, onion, and sweet potato. Cook until crispy, or until the onions are clear. This should take about 10 minutes.

Next, add the apples, thyme, garlic, and cinnamon. Cook the mixture for 30 seconds, and then add the chicken broth. Bring the mixture to a boil and cook for two and a half minutes, or until the broth has evaporated.

Add the chicken to the mixture, and cook for an additional two minutes, or until the chicken has warmed. Serve the skillet dish warm, and enjoy.

# Fruit Chutney with Salmon Curry

**Recipe Makes 4 Servings.**

Nutritional Breakdown Per Serving: 315 calories, 12 grams carbohydrates, 29 grams protein, 16 grams fat.

**Ingredients:**

4 salmon fillets

2 ½ tbsp. curry paste

2 tbsp. lime juice

**Chutney Ingredients:**

2 diced plums

1 diced nectarine

½ cup blueberries

½ tsp. cayenne pepper

1/3 cup diced onion

1 tsp. lime juice

Salt and pepper to taste

**Directions:**

Begin by stirring together the 2 ½ tbsp. curry paste with the initial 2 tbsp. lime juice in a baking dish. Position the salmon in the created mixture and then coat it. Cover the dish and allow it to refrigerate for 90 minutes.

Next, combine the chutney ingredients in a mixing bowl. Place the bowl in the refrigerator until serving time.

Next, preheat the oven to 425 degrees Fahrenheit. Uncover the salmon and allow it to bake for about 20 minutes.

Serve the salmon with the prepared chutney, and enjoy.

# Turkey and Essential Roasted Roots

**Recipe Makes 4 Servings.**

Nutritional Breakdown Per Serving: 215 calories, 15 grams carbohydrates, 28 grams protein, 5 grams fat.

**Ingredients:**

1 diced onion

3 diced carrots

1 diced yam

1 diced red pepper

1 diced beet

1 tbsp. olive oil

¾ pound ground turkey

½ tsp. basil

½ tsp. sage

½ tsp. sea salt

½ tsp. red pepper flakes

**Directions:**

Begin by preheating the oven to 375 degrees.

Next, slice and dice all the ingredients: onion, carrots, yams, red pepper, and beet. Position them together in a bowl. Next, place the ground turkey in the bowl, and stir well. Add all the spices to the bowl and stir well to create a perfectly assimilated mixture.

Next, position the mixture in a baking dish. Cover the baking dish and allow the roasted turkey to bake for twenty minutes. After twenty minutes, remove the top and bake the turkey for another fifteen minutes. Enjoy warm.

# Conclusion

I hope you have enjoyed this book and that it will help you to make a life-altering commitment, allowing you to embark upon a new "superfood" lifestyle. Superfoods are vibrant, pulsing with vitamins, minerals, and antioxidants, all of which help regulate your blood sugar, beat back against Type 2 diabetes, and other illnesses, such as cardiovascular disease, and live longer and better.

You cannot continue living as you have been, with a high-carbohydrate and high-sodium diet. It will destroy you if you don't change. Good luck on your new, type 2 diabetes journey, and remember that food is a powerful thing. Superfoods, namely, can change your very way of life.

Printed in Great
Britain
by Amazon